The Isolated Heart-Lung Preparation

P. H. Huisman and J. J. Schipperheyn
with technical assistance of
H. M. Kleijn
K. Kroll

1978
SPRINGER-SCIENCE+BUSINESS MEDIA, B.V.

In the course of some experiments made by me in conjunction with Dr. W.T. Sedgwick, on blood pressure in the coronary arteries of the heart, the fact was impressed upon me that the mammalian heart is no such fragile organ as one is usually inclined to assume, but possesses a very considerable power of bearing manipulation. On the other hand, I knew of various unsuccessful attempts to isolate the mammalian heart and study its physiology apart from the influence of extrinsic nerve centres, in a manner more or less less similar to the methods so frequently used for physiological investigations on the heart of a cold-blooded animal; the mammalian heart, however, always died before any observations could be made on it. Thinking over the apparent contradiction, it occurred to me that the essential difference probably lay in the coronary circulation; in the frog, as is well known, there are no coronary arteries or veins, the thin auricles and spongy ventricle being nourished by the blood flowing through the cardiac chambers, but in the mammal the thick-walled heart has a special circulatory system of its own and needs a steady flow through its vessels, and cannot be nourished (as appears to have been forgotten) by merely keeping up a stream through auricles and ventricles.

H. Newell Martin june 1881
from: Studies from the biological laboratory
of the John Hopkins University.

ISBN 978-90-247-2107-8 ISBN 978-94-009-9742-4 (eBook)
DOI 10.1007/978-94-009-9742-4

Originally published by MARTINUS NIJHOFF 1978

The development of an autoperfused canine heart-lung preparation formed part of a research project of the Interuniversity Cardiologic Institute, in which participated the Department of Cardiology of the State University of Leyden, the Netherlands.

The research was carried out in the Laboratory of Physiology, State University of Leyden. Design and manufacturing of most of the special equipment was done in the mechanical workshop (Head: Mr. R.P. de Graaf) and electronics department of this laboratory (Head: Mr. C.G. Wouters).

The publication of this book has been most generously supported by Astra Pharmaceutica B.V., to which the authors are truly grateful.

CONTENTS

1 INTRODUCTION

Need for isolated heart preparations

The study of cardiac function in a heart totally isolated from the body is required when one tries to relate properties of isolated cardiac muscle to heart function in the intact animal. Due to the fibre arrangement within the ventricular wall, the complexity of the spread of excitation, the presence of valves and the different problems related to relaxation and filling of the heart it is impossible to derive relations between pressure and flow throughout the cardiac cycle directly from length tension relationships which are obtained from studies on trabecula or papillary muscles. An isolated heart preparation is indispensable for the study of drug action on the heart. Only few drugs act solely on the heart, more often the vascular bed is influenced simultaneously and drug action cannot be ascertained due to the complex interaction of heart and vascular system.

History

The need for studies on isolated hearts has already been fully recognized about a century ago. Two different techniques to isolate hearts have evolved from that period which are still in use today, although in a modified version. In 1881 Newell Martin[12] described a functionally isolated heart-lung preparation in an open chest dog, in which an artificial haemodynamic resistor and a reservoir are inserted between aorta and caval veins, while the circulation to the body is interrupted. Loaded with an artificial impedance with a small priming volume, the so-called Starling resistor[8], the isolated heart-lung preparation of the dog served to

study the intrinsic contractile properties of the heart[8,15], cardiac metabolism[14], regulation of coronary flow[10] and the effects of various drugs.
In the Starling resistor the blood flows through a thin-walled collapsible tube, which is surrounded by a pressurized cylinder.

A second approach dates from 1895 when Langendorff developed a perfusion technique for the completely isolated rat's heart[9]. He demonstrated that oxygen can be dissolved in sufficient amounts in a saline solution to support a heart, which is perfused in the retrograde direction. Clearly it is of great advantage to use simple saline solutions as oxygenation of these solution does not create a problem and there is no need to include lungs in the preparation.

Both types of isolated heart preparations have their weak points and many investigators have tried to improve upon the original design. First, let us consider improvements to the classical Langendorff preparation. It requires a high coronary flow to compensate for the low oxygen content of the saline solution. It tends to develop edema which results from the low viscosity of the perfusion fluid and it obviously does not perform any external work because the left ventricle remains empty throughout the cardiac cycle. Mainly through the developed edema the mechanical properties of the muscle change continuously and effective experimentation is limited, depending on the limitations of the criteria for stability. Considerable improvement is obtained by addition of washed, usually bovine erythrocytes to the perfusion fluid. Coronary circulation and coronary venous PO_2 return to normal and viscosity can be increased, without hampering oxygen supply. A perfusion system, based on the Langendorff technique and which uses 'reconstituted blood' (containing washed erythrocytes and bovine serum albumine) allows for normal coronary flow regulation without the gradual increase of coronary vascular resistance caused by edema formation[3]. Another modification which makes the Langendorff preparation much more practicable is the addition of a reservoir, filled with perfusion fluid which has a constant pressure and which is connected to both the left atrium and the aorta through a system consisting of two one-way valves and an artificial vascular impedance[11]. The outflow from the coronary system thus is collected separately and usually not used for recirculation. In this way the left ventricle ejects and performs external work while the filling pressure and the aortic pressure can be controlled separately. A similar type of preparation has been developed for cat hearts by Elzinga[5].

As regards the original Starling heart-lung preparation,

it has not been subjected to so many modifications as has the Langendorff design. This book offers a description of a modified Starling preparation, which originally was developed for the purpose to study electrical activation of the ventricles and was later adapted to study valvular function and mechanical behaviour of the ventricles. Those studies require isolation of rather large hearts of about 250-450 g heart weight, pumping against normal pressure loads. For those hearts (generally from dogs and calves) the modified Langendorff technique is rather impractical, because it requires large quantities of perfusion fluid. The Starling preparation, however, offers distinct advantages over the modified Langendorff technique in this type of heart. The long period of stable mechanical performance and a high succes rate due to the simplicity of the method are among the advantages. An important benefit of this preparation is its use of whole, practically undiluted fresh blood with unchanged haemodynamic properties. Another important point is the conservation of the delicate relationship between pulmonary veins, left atrium and left ventricle which guarantees a normal filling pattern for the ventricle.

To correct for its weak points the original Starling preparation requires only a few minor modifications. First, the preparation should be taken completely out of the body to exclude external influences, especially from those of neuronal control. Secondly a servo controlled rollerpump should replace the reservoir at right atrial level for practical reasons, and a linear capillary resistor should be used instead of the Starling resistor so as to obtain more realistic pressure loads to the left ventricle. Detailed descriptions of modified Starling preparations are remarkably few in the recent literature[17].

Contents of this book

In this book a description is given of a Starling heart-lung preparation, designed and slightly modified with techniques and equipment available in 1977, 96 years after the original description by Newell Martin and his co-workers.

The description is probably of interest not only to physiologists and cardiologists but also to pharmacologists because of the preparation's unique facilities to study drug action. Especially the action of catecholamines and related compounds and of antiarrhythmic drugs are easily studied this way. The preparation may also be used to support other, even more delicate organs like brain or liver.

Our modified heart-lung preparation is completely isolated from the body and is suspended in a large, perspex box. It is attached with its aorta to a cannula from which it hangs freely in a humid, warm atmosphere. The pericardium may be removed but not necessarily so, if required the heart can be surrounded by water. An isolated heart can have a cardiac output of about 1.0 l/min/100 g against a mean aortic pressure of 70 mmHg, without catecholamine drive. A stable mechanical performance is maintained during a period of at least five hours. To adapt the preparation to certain specific studies many modifications of the technique are possible. A right heart bypass allows for coronary flow measurements and calculation of oxygen consumption. This adaptation also offers the possibility for opening the right ventricle for mapping of the spread of activation on the endocardium. The preparation can be altered with only minor modifications into a heart perfused in the retrograde fashion for similar studies on the endocardial surface of the left ventricle. Baan and his co-workers[1] have demonstrated that the preparation is an excellent starting point for a complete separation of the coronary from the systemic circulation. The main coronary arteries are more easily accessible and can be cannulated at leisure and thus in a more reliable way than with opened thorax only.

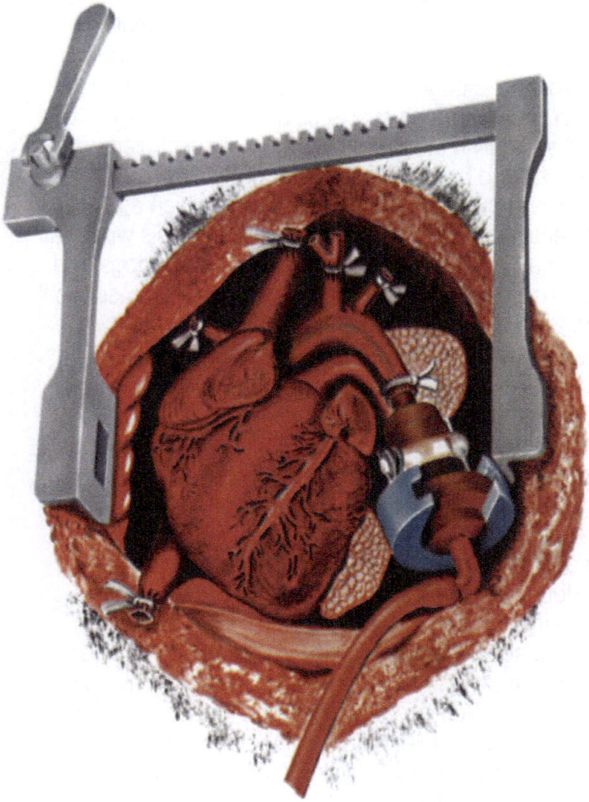

fig. 1

View into the opened thorax cavity when the heart has delivered all available blood to the reservoir. The azygos vein is ligated and cut before the cannula is inserted. The carotic arteries are closed off after the cannula's stop cock is opened. The caval veins are ligated and divided last, when the blood flow has almost stopped. The stop cock will be closed before the preparation is taken from the thorax.

---

2 THE ISOLATION PROCEDURE

The heart-lung preparation is usually obtained from large dogs of between 20-30 kg bodyweight. Calves can also be used. The required anaesthesia is achieved by administration of methadon with first a dose of droperidol. The usual dose is 2 mg/kg methadon i.v. and 1 mg/kg droperidol i.v.

Theoretically anaesthesia with volatile agents only should be preferred because these drugs will in due course of time disappear when the heart is isolated and the lungs are ventilated. For practical reasons, however, parenteral drugs

are chosen. The cardiac effects of the employed anaesthetic drugs are well documented and are known to be small[2,4]. After induction of anaesthesia the required depth is usually maintained long enough to complete the isolation procedure without an additional dose of anaesthetics. The animal is intubated and during thoracotomy is artificially ventilated with a mixture of air and oxygen. A capnograph (Godart) measures end-expiratory PCO_2 levels from which a proper level of ventilation is set. A mild metabolic acidosis will be a rather typical finding in methadon anaesthesia in dogs and in order to compensate for this an isotonic $NaHCO_3$-solution is infused of which usually 200-300 ml is required.
The exact quantity is determined by measuring the bicarbonate concentration in the arterial blood.

Thoracotomy is performed by a midline incision through the sternum. The heart and the major blood vessels are exposed, the pericardium is usually kept intact.
The azygos vein is ligated and cut between ligatures.
Both the caval veins, the carotid artieries and the descending aorta are subsequently ligated but not closed as yet. Heparin is given (200 mg i.v.) and a wide bore cannula, inner diameter 10 mm, is next inserted into the descending aorta. The carotid arteries should be closed after cannulation (fig. 1). Closing of the carotid arteries prior to cannulation is likely to cause damage to the heart. The aortic cannula, which later in time is to be used to connect the preparation to the perfusion system, will temporarily be connected to a Starling resistor. Through this resistor the heart can pump arterial blood into the reservoir of the perfusion system, while a proper perfusion pressure for the coronary arteries is maintained. The perfusion pressure is usually set at about 50 mmHg. The caval veins are closed and divided after the aortic flow has stopped completely and the heart is emptied by releasing the pressure from the Starling resistor. The perfusion system does not require a priming volume. Lungs are next inflated and the trachea is cross-clamped and cut. The aortic cannula is closed with a stop cock and disconnected from the Starling resistor. At that moment a short period of myocardial ischemia is bound to occur. Within this period the heart-lung preparation is taken from the thorax and transferred to the perfusion box. In the box, the arterial blood is already circulating and retrograde perfusion of the coronary arteries, once the heart is connected to the box, is started immediately. Perfusion pressure is set at about 75 mmHg by the pressure inside the Starling resistor. Ventilation of the lungs should be continued with an air, oxygen, carbondioxide mixture. Venous blood returning to the empty thorax cavity is collected. This blood contains very little oxygen and is severely acidotic. A sodium

bicarbonate solution is therefore added and the blood is filtered before it is added to the arterial blood which circulates in the perfusion system. A wide bore cannula is connected to the right atrium, through the inferior caval vein. The retrograde perfusion of the coronary arteries is next changed into a normal antegrade heart-lung perfusion by pumping the blood from the reservoir into the right atrium. Antegrade perfusion usually improves the condition of the preparation, it increases pulmonary perfusion and facilitates oxygen uptake. A rapid transition from retrograde to antegrade perfusion probably is very important because it protects the coronary system from accidental embolization. We therefore try to keep the period of retrograde perfusion as short as possible. After addition of venous blood the total of circulating blood amounts to 1500 to 2000 ml, depending on the size of the animal. The pericardium can be kept intact, but can be removed to expose the heart for electrical measurements. During the isolation procedure we prefer to leave it intact.

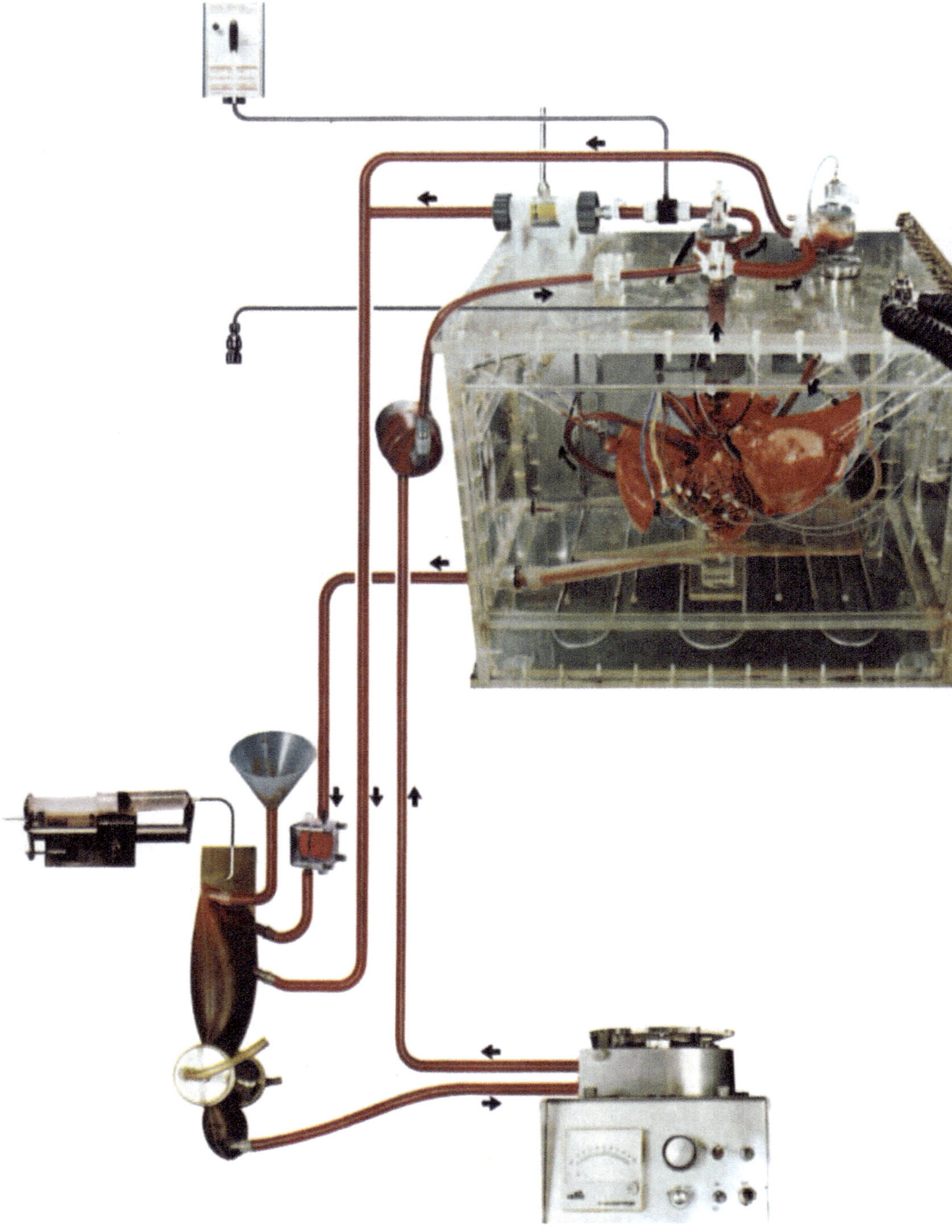

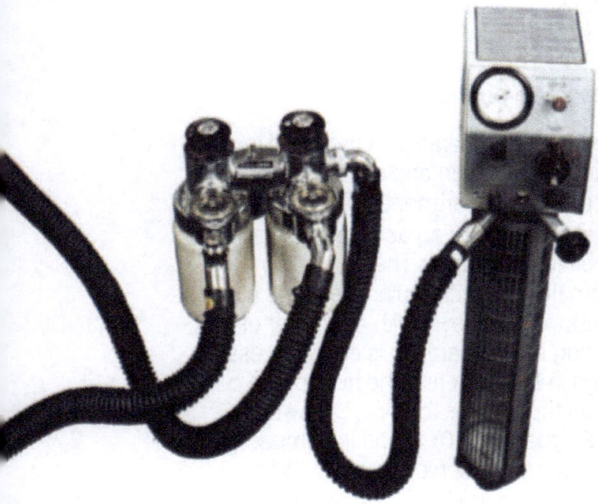

fig. 2

Perfusion box with ventilator and rollerpump.
Blood flows from the reservoir to the rollerpump, through a filter to a valve placed centrally in the top of the box. If used for antegrade perfusion the blood passes directly to a second valve, placed more to the right. From there it can either flow back to the reservoir or through a long cannula to the right atrium. Blood flow from the left ventricle runs through an electromagnetic flow probe and Starling resistor back to the reservoir. Blood leaking from the heart is collected in a dish placed under the heart and is filtered before returned to the reservoir. An infusion pump is used for supply of glucose, insulin and heparin.

3 PERFUSION BOX

Retrograde and antegrade perfusion

The isolated heart-lung preparation is mounted in a large perspex perfusion box (Design and construction, Mechanical Workshop of the Department of Physiology, State University Leyden), which during actual measurements is completely closed off from room air. The heart-lung preparation hangs from the aortic cannula. The lungs are supported and fixed above heart level with a number of sutures. During mounting the preparation is easily accessible through large openings in the back and the front of the box. A blood reservoir is situated outside the box, below table-top level (Polystan A/S, type HL 290). Blood is pumped (Collin-Trans Omega) from the reservoir through a filter (Pall-Ultipor Blood filter 3/8") to the top of the box. It enters the box from above through a large two way valve placed in de middle of the top. Blood can flow either to the aorta or to the right atrium. The valve serves to switch rapidly from retrograde to antegrade perfusion (fig. 2 and 3, see also enclosure at the back of the book).

In the retrograde perfusion mode, the blood flow to the aorta is shunted back to the reservoir through a Starling resistor. The air pressure inside it determines the perfusion pressure of the coronary system. In antegrade perfusion blood enters the right atrium and the Starling resistor serves as an external impedance to the left ventricle. In this way the heart is self perfused, the pump is there only to compensate for hydrostatic pressure differences in the system. It can be used to govern ventricular filling. Set at constant volumetric flow, the output of the pump exactly equals aortic flow in steady state condition. Left atrial pressure rises to a level necessary to produce an enddiastolic filling of the left ventricle sufficiently high to eject the required flow against a given aortic pressure. A servo-control of the pump (Design: Electronics Dept. Laboratory for Physiology, State University Leyden) is used to adjust inflow in order to keep left atrial pressure constant under varying aortic pressure loads.

The impedance of a Starling resistance differs greatly from the peripheral impedance to the vascular bed of the intact circulation. To study isolated hearts under more 'physiological' conditions an artificial impedance of the type developed by Westerhof et al[22] can be used. Perfusion, however, is first started with a conventional Starling resistance and in a later stage aortic flow will be switched to the Westerhof resistance.

Right heart bypass technique

The perfusion box can also be used for a variant mode of antegrade perfusion: the so called right heart bypass technique. A cannula is inserted into the left pulmonary artery and the vessel is ligated proximally. The flow from the perfusion pump to the right atrium is then dilivered directly into the left lung through this cannula. The right pulmonary artery caries mixed venous blood from the coronary system only.

This allows one to measure coronary flow and mixed coronary venous oxygen saturation (Edwards Flow-directed oxymeter catheter no. 01-110-6F and Physio Control In-vivo oxymeter) from which myocardial oxygen consumption can be calculated.

With the right heart bypass technique it is also possible to open the right ventricle for electrical measurements at the endocardial surface. The blood flowing from the opened cavity is collected in a dish placed under the preparation. It should be filtered before returned to the reservoir. Similar measurements can be performed on the left side by opening the ventricle while the coronary arteries are perfused retrogradely. Aortic valves remain competent and the already reoxygenated coronary blood is collected and returned to the reservoir after filtering.

Pressure lines are inserted, usually in the left atrium and the left ventricle, the pulmonary artery and aorta (connected to Statham P23Db pressure transducers). Aortic flow is measured by an electromagnetic flowmeter (Skalar-Transflow 601), the probe of which is placed about 5 cm above the aortic valves (fig. 4). If the right heart bypass technique is applied a perivascular probe is attached to the right pulmonary artery to measure coronary flow, and a fibre optic catheter is inserted into the

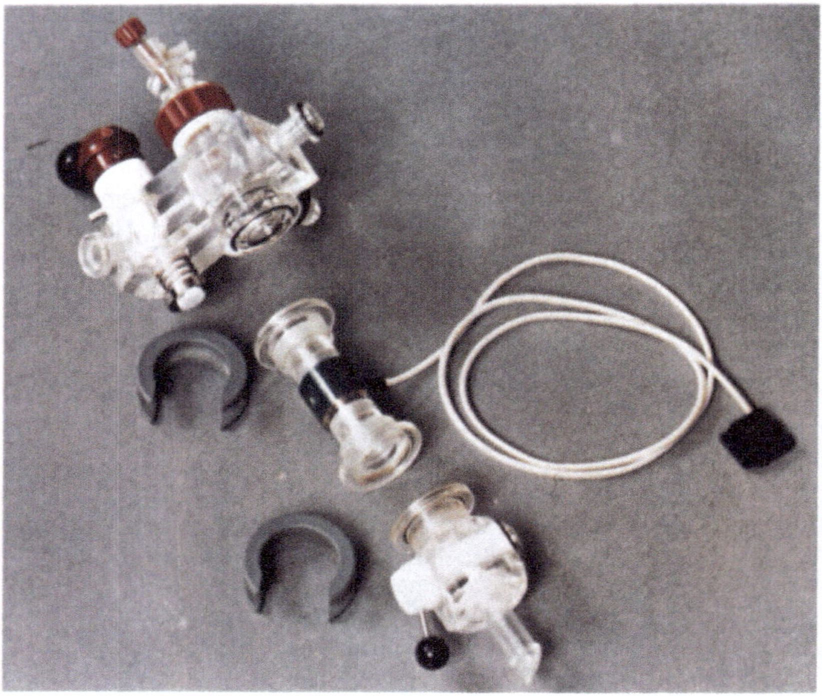

fig. 4
Aortic cannula, electromagnetic flow probe and central valve with quick-release connectors.

pulmonary main stem for continuous oxymetry.

Humidity and temperature

Mixed venous coronary blood is sampled for chemical analysis and for off-line calibration of the oxymeter. The bottom of the perfusion box is filled with water up to 4 cm. The water is heated by a heat exchanger fed from a hot-water supply (Tamson-Holland). Air bubbles through the water with some force to agitate the air inside the box, this increases humidity to about full saturation. Blood in the reservoir is heated by passing it through a heat exchanger. Care is taken to match the blood temperatures exactly to the temperature inside the box. This is achieved by using a double feed-back control (Design: Electronical Department, Laboratory of Physiology, State University Leyden) on both the hot water supplies to the heat exchangers in the blood reservoir and to the perfusion box. Opening of windows in the perfusion box should be avoided during measurements. Exposure of the heart to ambient temperature will cool off the epicardial surface of the heart. As a result temperature differences of 2-3° C between cavity and epicardial surface will arise. There is little doubt that even a slight temperature gradient across the myocardial wall greatly influences electrical as well as mechanical phenomena of the heart.

Ventilation and pacing

Ventilation of the lungs does not create large problems. The condition of the lungs is preserved best if ventilation is kept at 2-3 $l min^{-1}$ depending on the size of the lungs. (Monaghan 300 D/M ventilator). This level of ventilation is much higher than is really needed for gas exchange. To avoid a drop of carbon dioxide content because of overventilation some carbon dioxide should be added to the respiratory gas mixture. The carbon dioxide partial pressure is set at about 35 mmHg by means of a capnograph (Godart). The condition of the lungs is best preserved if the oxygen fraction is kept below 30%.
The arterial PO_2 in the system is usually set at about 150 mmHg.

Routinely two electrodes are sutured on to the heart. One is attached to the right atrium, the other to the apex to obtain electrocardiographic signals. Also a set of pacing electrodes is sutured on the right atrium; 0.2 mm diameter at 2 mm distance. A fixed heart rate is achieved by overpacing the sinus node. At a temperature of 38.5° C the spontaneous sinus node frequency is about 130-140 min^{-1} and the artificial pacemaker is therefore set at about 150 min^{-1}.

4 CARDIAC METABOLISM, ELECTROLYTE SHIFTS AND ACID-BASE PROBLEMS

Blood freshly taken from the animal contains a sufficient amount of glucose, and free fatty acids (FFA) to supply the working heart with energy for up to one hour. Possibly, in addition some glucose and FFA are released from intracardiac stores. However, this contribution is probably small when suitable glucose concentrations are maintained. Cholesterol and triglycerides are not metabolized and their concentration in the circulating blood remains stable throughout. After one hour of perfusion time, the FFA content of the blood has fallen to very low values and cellular metabolism has probably shifted completely to glucose breakdown. The preparation then requires a constant infusion of glucose, to which a sufficient amount of insulin should be added. The amount needed varies with heart weight, temperature and workload, but 0.02 $mmol.h^{-1}$ glucose for each 100 gr heart weight given in a 10% solution is sufficient to keep glucose concentration between 5 and 15 $mmol.l^{-1}$. By measuring the glucose content of the blood at regular intervals the glucose consumption of the preparation can be calculated. It is known that aerobic breakdown of glucose requires 6 mmol of oxygen for each mmol, that is 155 ml at 38.5° C. During the first hour of perfusion the heart consumes more oxygen than needed for its glucose consumption, but later glucose and oxygen uptake match exactly. Obviously, when circulating FFA have been used up, glucose forms the sole source of energy and FFA release from internal stores does not significantly contribute to energy supply under these conditions.

In blood perfused preparations, anaerobic glucose metabolism and formation of lactic acid are always signs of

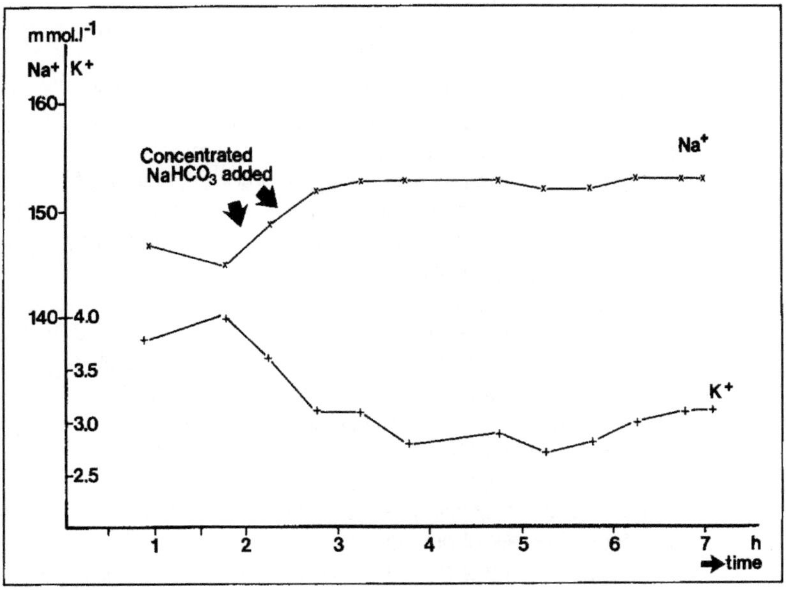

fig. 5

Sodium and potassium concentration of the circulating blood during six hours of perfusion. The heart is isolated one hour after the start of the experiment. To correct for metabolic acidosis an 8.4 % $NaHCO_3$-solution is added, as a result the sodium concentration increases. Potassium concentration decreases for two hours because of a cell inward shift of these ions. Later the potassium concentration increases due to haemolysis.

---

insufficient perfusion in some part of the heart usually caused by accidental embolization of the coronary system. Lactate concentration drops rapidly after isolation and after initial correction of metabolic acidosis further addition of bicarbonate ions is not necessary. In our experience the addition of lactate or pyruvate to the perfusion fluid does not improve the mechanical performance of the heart. Electrolyte concentrations usually vary a little during perfusion. This is due in part to the necessary initial addition of sodium bicarbonate, but also to mechanical haemolysis and to potassium shifts induced by the enhanced glucose metabolism and correction of acidosis. The time course of Na^+ and K^+ concentrations in a typical experiment is shown in fig. 5. Initial correction of metabolic acidosis is done by adding 15 ml of an 8.4% $NaHCO_3$ solution. This causes a slight increase of the Na^+ concentration. The correction of acidosis in the presence of an enhanced glucose metabolism is followed by a significant cell inward shift of K^+-ions and a reduction of the K^+-concentration from 4.0 to 2.8 mmol.l^{-1}. After this initial drop the K^+–

concentration rises slowly. During perfusion some degree of haemolysis is unavoidable and K^+-ions released from erythrocytes can be expected to increase the K^+–concentration gradually during perfusion. The increase is small however, because canine red blood cells contain a relatively low concentration of potassium (10 $mmol.l^{-1}$) compared to human erythrocytes (95 $mmol.l^{-1}$). In view of the observed changes of Na^+ and K^+ concentrations correction of metabolic acidosis should be completed early, to reduce potassium shifts during measurements.
The resulting increase of the sodium concentration has probably some influence on cardiac function. To avoid this, isotonic bicarbonate solution should be used (1.4% solution of $NaHCO_3$) and appropriate amounts of $CaCl_2$ and KCl should be added. The cell inward shift of K^+-ions requires the extra addition of KCl, to correct for the resulting hypokaliaemia. Proper correction of acidosis and hypokaliaemia improves mechanical function of the heart, it reduces the rate of development of haemolysis and pulmonary edema and greatly reduces the incidence of arrhythmias.

5 HAEMOLYSIS AND PULMONARY EDEMA

Pumping and filtering blood, and even exposure to air inevitably causes mechanical haemolysis to occur. The isolated heart-lung preparation is perfused with recirculating blood and its survival is limited by mechanical haemolysis and related processes. Haemolysis increases the viscosity of the blood, but also releases adenosine diphosphate (ADP) from red blood cells. ADP has a vasodilating effect on the coronary system, it also stimulates the aggregation of circulating platelets. ADP release is the most important factor contributing to the rapid disappearance of platelets form the circulating blood. Platelet aggregates are probably involved in the formation of vasoactive substances related to prostaglandines from lipoproteins. These substances exert a dilating effect on capillaries, both in the coronary system[6] and in the lungs[7] and may promote the development of edema by increasing the permeability of the capillary wall. In the heart, dilatation of myocardial capillaries interferes with coronary autoregulation, which limits the heart's ability to withstand extreme aortic pressure values. In the lungs capillary dilatation decreases the ventilation perfusion ratio which disturbes to a degree oxygenation. The increased permeability of the pulmonary capillaries leads to the eventual development of pulmonary edema, even if the lungs are raised above the heart level. This cannot be prevented by positive pressure ventilation.

The process of haemolysis should be carefully monitored by measuring the free haemoglobine content of the circulating blood or by determination of the concentration of free lactate dehydrogenase (LDH) in the

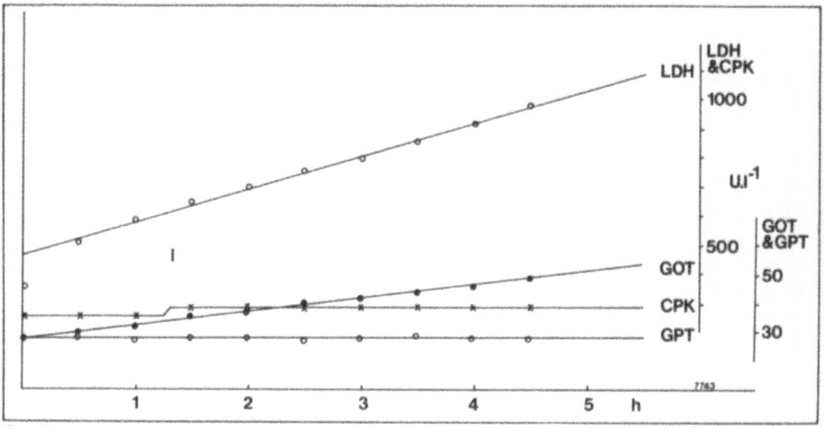

fig. 6

Enzym concentrations during a 4.5 hour perfusion period. Vertical bar indicates the insertion of a needle electrode into the septum.

---

plasma. From figure 6 it follows that the rate of haemolysis is fairly constant for a period up to five hours. After five hours of perfusion, the rate of haemolysis is usually found to increase slightly. From the data presented it follows that about 100 $U.l^{-1}$ LDH are released per hour, all from damaged erythrocytes. Concommittantly the concentration of glutamic oxaloacetic transaminase (GOT) is found to increase with about 4 $U.l^{-1}$ per hour. This GOT release is from blood cells, which in dogs contain a small quantity of this enzyme. The stable concentration of both creatine phosphokinase (CPK) and glutamic pyruvic transaminase (GPT), two enzymes present in canine cardial tissue, demonstrates the absence of myocardial cell destruction. The small step-wise increase of CPK content after one hour reflects the insertion of an electrode needle. The initial rise of the LDH concentration is explained by some damage done to pulmonary tissues when the lungs are fixed above the heart.
Release of 100 $U.l^{-1}$ LDH corresponds roughly to the destruction of 0.5% of the circulating red cells and the release of 3 $g.l^{-1}$ of haemoglobine. Mechanical haemolysis can be kept down to this level by a careful design of the system in avoiding sharp edges. Only one filter is used (Pall-Ultipor 3/8") in the pathway between rollerpump and preparation and exposure of blood to air is avoided as far as possible. Formation of thrombocyte aggregation is slowed down if non-thrombogenic materials are used for tubes and valves. The rate of mechanical haemolysis is greatly increased by changing the temperature, or pH of the blood. Dilution of the blood with saline solution also seems

to increase the rate of this process. Moreover, there is little doubt that synthesis and release of vasodilating substances and the development of edema are caused not only by mechanical haemolysis, but also by mechanical damage to other tissues in the heart and lungs.
Adverse effects can be noted from extensive handling of the lung, squeezing of the heart, over-inflation of the lungs, electrical defibrillation of the heart, periods of hypoxia, and extreme haemodynamic conditions.
Mechanical haemolysis and release of vasoactive substances significantly interfere with electrical and mechanical performance of the heart, only after four or five hours of perfusion. Interference with coronary autoregulation is reflected in a gradual increase of both coronary flow and oxygen saturation of coronary venous blood, which does not affect mechanical cardiac performance however, unless extreme pressure loads are imposed upon the heart. The reduction of ventilation perfusion ratio in the lungs causes a gradual decline of arterial PO_2, but oxygen content of the blood is not critically decreased during the first five hours of perfusion (fig. 7). Vasodilation and damage to the capillary wall cannot be completely avoided if recirculated whole blood is used for perfusion of the

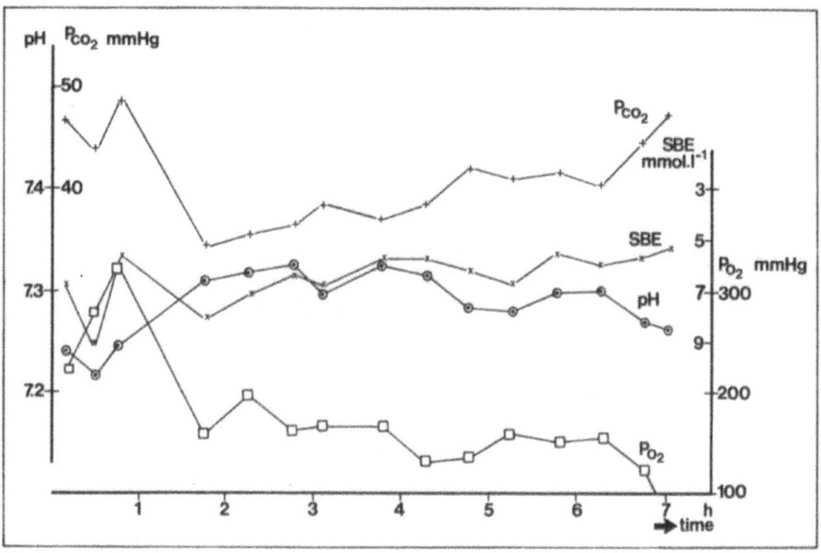

fig. 7

Bloodgas concentrations, bicarbonate levels and pH during a seven hour perfusion period.
PCO_2 and PO_2 are predominantly determined by the composition of the respiratory gas mixture, which is corrected after 1.5 hours, just after correction of metabolic acidosis.
Bicarbonate concentration is raised after one hour by adding a concentrated $NaHCO_3$-solution. After 6.5 hours of perfusion pulmonary edema developed.

preparation, but it can be limited so that myocardial functions continue sufficiently long to complete a relevant study.

The use of reconstituted blood, containing saline solution, washed erythrocytes and bovine albumine as developed by Duvelleroy[3] for perfusion of rat's heart is probably advantageous, because one or several factors involved in the synthesis of vasodilating substances seem to be missing. The complete absence of thrombocytes in artificial perfusion media however, induces formation of petecchia and occasionally confluent haemorrhages in the myocardium.

6 ELECTRICAL MEASUREMENTS

The canine heart in the isolated heart-lung preparation as a rule settles to a highly regular sinus rhythm, its frequency depending mainly on temperature and up to a slight degree on right atrial filling pressure.
At a temperature of 38.5° C, a common body temperature for a dog, sinus node frequency in the isolated heart is about 130-140 per minute, which is considerably faster than commonly found in intact dogs under resting condition. This discrepancy is believed to be caused by a high vagal nerve tonus in the intact animal. Also, the distinct respiratory arrhythmia commonly observed in resting dogs seems to be centrally mediated since it is not found in the isolated heart, although right atrial pressure varies a little with respiration. The absence of a steady background of vagal nerve activity in the isolated preparation can be demonstrated by adding atropine. This exerts no measurable effect.
Blocking of sympathetic nerve activity by propranolol one hour after perfusion fails to affect node frequency as well as mechanical properties of the isolated heart. This demonstrates that resting activity of sympathetic nerves has died out at that time, and that the concentration of circulating catecholamines has fallen to very low values.

Intra-atrial conduction is not influenced by the isolation procedure, as can be judged from the duration of the P-wave and the pattern of activation. Atrio ventricular conduction in isolated hearts is usually somewhat slower than in the intact animal, as can be judged from the PR-interval, which varies between 120 and 140 ms, compared to 90 and 110 ms in the intact dog at the same temperature.

This difference is insufficiently explained, the disappearance of the catecholamine-drive on the AV-node present in the intact animal may be involved, also changes in atrial pressure may play a role. The increased PR-interval is caused by a slowing of nodal conduction, conduction along the Hisbundle is found to be unchanged.

Intraventricular conduction along the Purkinje fibers of the bundle and its ramifications and along myocardial fibers is not affected by the isolation procedure.
The duration of the QRS-complex is therefore not changed, provided that the heart's temperature remains the same. The duration of the QRS-complex at 38.5° C varies between 45-50 ms from one heart to another. Exposing the heart to room temperature which cools superficial myocardial layers increases QRS-duration considerably.

Artificial stimulation of the isolated heart can be achieved by overpacing the sinus node activity through a pair of silver wire electrodes (surface area 0.10 mm^2, 2 mm apart), preferably sutured on the right atrial epicardial surface, close to the position of the sinus node. Artificial pacing at low frequencies requires blocking of AV-conduction or destruction of nodal tissue[21]. Artificial pacing at constant frequency is necessary in all studies on conduction, to exclude the effect of heart rate on impulse propagation.
Recording of atrial or ventricular electrical activity can most conveniently be done by using metal wire electrodes, surface area between 0.03 and 0.5 mm^2. Silver, stainless steel or platinum is to be preferred to other metarials if stable recording conditions are required lasting many hours. Epicardial electrodes are best hooked onto an elastic mesh, which is fixed around the heart. In this way one avoids damage to the muscle. Plunged electrodes, both single wire or multiple electrode needles, cause some unavoidable damage to the heart muscle, as seen by the appearance of large ST-elevations, immediately after insertion. The extent of the damage can be deduced from sequential determinations of CPK concentration in the circulating blood (fig. 6). One plunged needle electrode 1.2 mm in diameter, inserted 36 mm deep into the septum releases about 50 U of CPK. As myocardial tissue contains approximately 1000 U of CPK per gram, the amount of damage by one needle can be estimated to be about 50 mg. Assuming cell destruction to be homogeneously distributed, the damage extents to a depth of 0.37 mm from the needle surface. Injury potentials usually disappear within one hour, because intercalated discs between damaged and healthy cells seal off and isolate the damaged part electrically.
Most studies on electrical properties of the heart can be performed on simple preparations like the exposed heart in

an anaesthetized animal or the retrogradely perfused non-working heart. But for some studies however, the isolated heart-lung preparation is indispensable. The primary advantage of the isolated heart-lung preparation lies in the excellent control over the haemodynamic relationships in and around the heart, which can be achieved without interference of the autonomic nervous system.
The preparation is ideally suited to study the effect of acute pressure and volume changes on electrical behaviour of the heart. Some electrical phenomena in the heart are very insensitive to haemodynamic changes especially intramural spread of activation. Voltage distributions in the heart during the P-wave or the QRS complex changes when intra ventricular volume is increased, but the duration of these phenomena and the time of arrival of the activation wave-front at different positions remains identical. Also, aortic pressure changes do not affect the spread of myocardial activation. Atrial pressure does have an influence on nodal activity in the isolated heart-lung preparation like in other types of isolated heart preparations. Sinus frequency is found to increase with atrial pressure, while AV-nodal conduction delay time increases. This effect has not been completely investigated, especially when left atrial pressure is increased independent from right atrial pressure as in the right heart bypass technique. The purely mechanical influence of atrial wall stretch on nodal tissue seems to explain the observed changes in heart rate and conduction only in part.

Another interesting field which is opened up by the isolated heart-lung technique is the study of repolarization of the heart. ST-segments and T-waves are notoriously sensitive to changes in the condition of the preparation, especially to pressure and flow relations but also to catecholamine levels and vagal and sympathetic nerve activity.
Repolarization is not a stable, reproducible phenomenon in the exposed intact heart. Only with permanently implanted electrodes stable recordings have been obtained[19].
In retrogradely perfused preparations the repolarization of the ventricle is known to be far more sensitive to gradual developing edema than the depolarization process and studies of repolarization performed in these preparations have rendered conflicting results. Preliminary studies in the isolated heart-lung preparation have demonstrated that the shape of ST-segments and T-wave may remain identical for at least four hours if haemodynamic conditions are stable. It seems likely that, next to the temperature distribution and heart rate at least three different parameters exert some influence on repolarization: end diastolic pressure, aortic pressure and oxygen supply to the heart. It is not clear as

yet whether the pronounced changes induced by hypoxia result from a direct effect of reduced oxygen tension on membrane properties only or also from the influence of locally released catecholamines. Adrenergic blocking drugs will reduce the observed changes which indicates that local catecholamine-release probably in the development of ST changes is more important than is usually assumed. Another intriguing point is that the effects of high aortic pressure cannot be separated completely from anoxic or ischemic effects, as high aortic pressures tend to induce subendocardial ischemia, especially if coronary autoregulation is partly compromised by circulating vasodilating agents. Further investigations, especially with high dosages of adrenergic blocking agents may be able to separate these different phenomena.

7 HAEMODYNAMICS

Isolation of the heart-lung preparation from the body and the replacement of the systemic blood vessels by an artificial peripheral impedance does not leave the haemodynamic relations in the heart completely unchanged. The filling pressure which is required to pump out a cardiac output of two litres per minute against a mean arterial blood pressure of 70 mmHg is considerably lower in the isolated preparation than in the heart in situ. The end-diastolic shape of the ventricle is different and the waveforms of both the aortic pressure and flow are changed by the isolation procedure. These discrepancies between isolated and in-situ hearts require some further analysis.

If the isolated preparation is operated at constant aortic flow by keeping the rollerpump at a fixed output level, left atrial pressure at a given heart rate is determined by the aortic pressure and the contractile state of the left ventricle. At a given aortic pressure level and constant flow the left ventricular filling pressure thus serves as a measure of left ventricular performance. For one litre per minute aortic flow and 70 mmHg mean aortic pressure mean left atrial pressure should be between −1.5 and −0.5 mmHg. (0-reference at mid-atrial level between inferior and superior caval vein). Higher values indicate damage to the myocardial wall usually incurred during isolation.
An increase of aortic pressure is met by a rise of left ventricular end diastolic pressure and left atrial pressure. At a mean aortic pressure of about 140 mmHg, a critical afterload level is reached, which cannot be overcome by further increase of left atrial pressure. Above this critical

level left atrial pressure rises steeply and the functioning of the preparation is in danger from rapid developing pulmonary edema and pooling of all circulating blood in the lungs and right heart. This critical aortic pressure level is considerably lower than the pressure levels found in the intact circulation when peripheral resistance is increased considerably. It should be kept in mind however, that the isolated heart is forced to maintain a constant aortic flow and that it is deprived of any catecholamine drive.

The low atrial pressure of the isolated preparation compared to the intact heart at similar flow and pressure values is not explained by the removal of the pericardium. At normal pressure and flow values, removal of the pericardium has very little effect on left atrial pressure indicating that it does not influence end-diastolic compliance significantly at low end-diastolic pressure. The low atrial pressure is probably completely explained by the presence of a large hydrostatic pressure difference in the isolated heart, when surrounded by air. The absence of

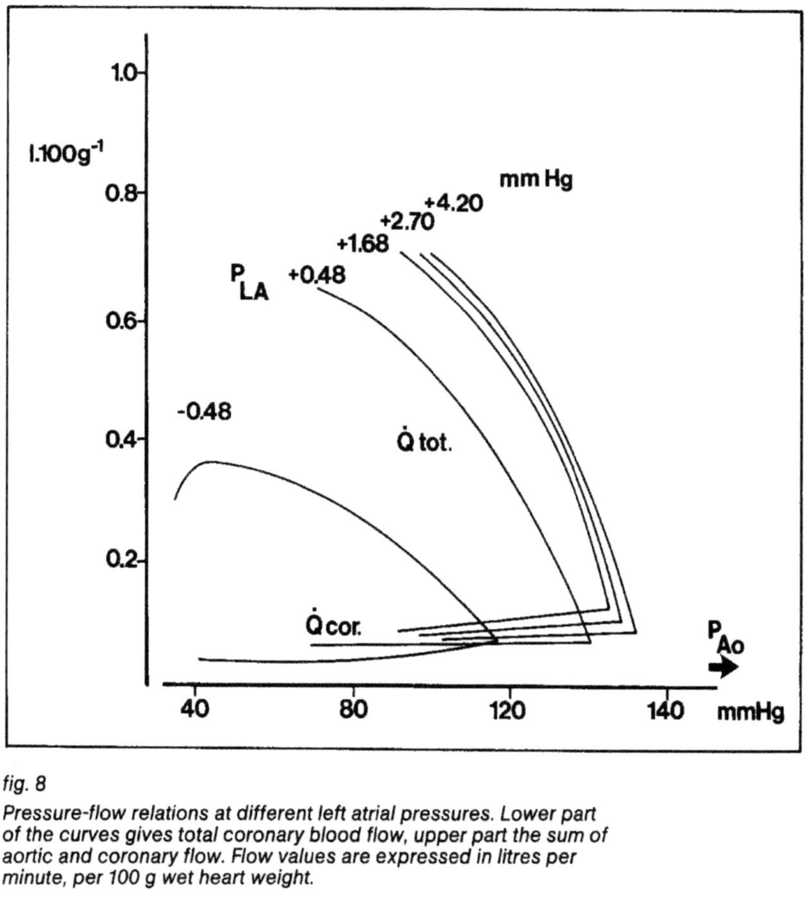

fig. 8

Pressure-flow relations at different left atrial pressures. Lower part of the curves gives total coronary blood flow, upper part the sum of aortic and coronary flow. Flow values are expressed in litres per minute, per 100 g wet heart weight.

lungs and mediastinal structures around the heart also accounts for the somewhat pearshaped appearance of the heart during diastole. Apical regions appear to be stretched considerably more during diastole than areas close to the valves. It should be kept in mind that because of the induced inhomogeneity of the initial fiber length, the rate of pressure development is influenced. The contribution of early activated apical regions is enhanced and that of late activated regions of the outflow tract is reduced compared to the intact situation. Surrounding the heart and lungs with saline solution abolishes the hydrostatic pressure differences and reduces the inhomogeneity of initial fibre length along the main axis of the heart, but it does not restore the normal filling pattern and shape of the heart during diastole completely. This can probably only be achieved by immersion of the preparation in a medium mimmicking the mechanical properties of pulmonary tissue. So, the ventricular filling is altered, not only in completely isolated hearts but also in the in-situ exposed heart with opened thorax, mainly by the removal of the surrounding tissue. This should be kept in mind, when interpreting results obtained in such a situation.

More discrepancies between isolated and in-situ hearts are revealed by operating the preparation at constant left atrial pressure. An increase of mean aortic pressure in this mode is met by a decrease of aortic flow. To achieve constant left atrial pressure independent from aortic pressure, feed-back control on the systemic flow is superior to the traditional technique in which the left atrium is connected to a constant pressure reservoir. Interference with atrial and valvular function and the relatively high haemodynamic resistance of the connection between reservoir and atrium disturb the filling of the left ventricle. The time course of left atrial pressure is changed by such a technique and is made to resemble the shape of a left atrial pressure curve in cases of combined mitral valvular disease. Flow rates at a given left atrial and aortic pressure combination are usually considerably lower if a constant pressure reservoir is used, instead of a feed-back control on systemic flow.

Pressure-flow diagrams at different left atrial pressures, obtained with systemic flow control are demonstrated in fig. 8. Application of the right heart bypass technique allows for simultaneous measurement of total coronary flow and aortic flow. From this diagram classical function curves of the heart can be derived by plotting flow at constant aortic pressure as a function of left atrial pressure. The function curve in the heart from which fig. 8 data is obtained has a rising phase which extends from −0.7 to about +1.7 mmHg, further increase of left atrial pressure produces very little increase of flow. This steep rising phase is typical for an

isolated heart surrounded by air. A plateau is reached at about 4 mmHg, a declining phase of the function curve is usually not found, up to 15 mmHg. Higher left atrial pressures, above 15 mmHg cannot be investigated fully because of development of pulmonary edema. Cardiac output rises if aortic pressure is lowered, it has the tendency to approach a constant level at mean aortic pressure levels below 50 mmHg.
Further reduction of aortic pressure eventually leads to insufficient coronary perfusion. Below a critical minimal perfusion pressure overt signs of ischemia develop and cardiac output is no longer maintained. This critical pressure can be as low as 25 mmHg in some hearts.
Its level seems to depend largely on the effectiveness of coronary autoregulatory processes. The minimal perfusion pressure tends to go up, during perfusion while autoregulation of the coronary system becomes progressively impeded.

At the higher end of the aortic pressure range, cardiac output eventually equals coronary flow. Mean aortic pressure at this point is the so-called cross-clamp pressure. It may reach values up to 160 mmHg, depending on the condition of coronary autoregulation. In some hearts stable cross-clamped perfusion cannot be achieved.
On approaching cross-clamp pressure in these hearts, signs of subendocardial ischemia develop and myocardial function deteriorates rapidly. Signs of ischemia at high aortic pressure develop only in hearts in which the coronary system is already dilated due to a compromised autoregulation.
In healthy, freshly isolated hearts the cross-clamped situation may be maintained without signs of ischemia, but high aortic pressure exerts harmful influence on coronary autoregulation also in these hearts. When pressure is returned to normal coronary flow remains excessively elevated, recovery is extremely slow and never complete.

The behaviour of the autoperfused heart at both extremely high and extremely low aortic pressures is of much interest for its clinical counterpart. The deleterious effects of aortic cross-clamping are well-known in cardiac surgery. Exposure of the heart to high blood pressure is bound to have adverse effects in almost all cardiac emergencies, especially those resulting from coronary artery disease. An injurious effect on coronary autoregulation ultimately leading to progressive subendocardial ischemia and infarction seems to be the basic mechanism involved.

Lowering of arterial blood pressure, on the other hand, is reported to be beneficial in patients suffering from acute myocardial infarction or otherwise endangered myocardial function. A sufficiently high perfusion pressure should be maintained, not only for vital organs like the brain and kidneys, but also for the heart itself. Knowledge about its critical level and the effects of different drugs on this level would provide important information for the further development of blood pressure lowering therapy.

In studies on mechanical behaviour the isolated heart should preferably be loaded with an artificial impedance which closely matches the input impedance of the natural vascular system. In the classical design used by Starling and his co-workers the peripheral impedance comprised a Starling resistor and a capacitor, made from an air-filled tube[8]. The simplicity of the design and its low priming volume are an important advantage, but the input impedance of such a system is quite unlike that of the systemic circulation and the pressure-flow relationship is highly nonlinear. Stenosed tubes or pressure reservoirs do not form a proper load for a heart for similar reasons.

According to the design by Westerhof et al[22] of a hydraulic analog impedance for an isolated cat heart a three element windkessel was constructed for the dog heart-lung preparation. The resistors consist of many capillary tubes in parallel, the capacitor is an air-filled chamber, separated from the blood by a thin membrane (fig. 9). The canine heart-lung preparation requires a capillary bed much larger than the cat heart, also because of the higher viscosity of whole blood the number of capillaries should be larger than in the Westerhof design. A good linear pressure-flow relationship could be obtained from a capillary resistor made from five commercially available artificial kidneys (Cordis 2.5 D) (fig. 10).
The proximal resistor is made from a polythene slab with 2500 holes 0.5 mm in diameter.
The value of the resistor can be changed in a stepwise fashion by closing off a number of kidneys. As soon as a kidney is closed, circulation through the capillaries is maintained with a separate roller-pump to avoid obstruction and changes in temperature and composition of the blood. The mantles of the kidneys are circulated with a buffered saline solution at proper temperature. To avoid a loss of water from the blood the pressure in the mantle should be kept at approximately the same level as the aortic pressure.

The linear properties of the capillary resistor allow for computation of input impedance and source impedance and the use of Fourier Analysis of aortic pressure and flow to calculate total external power of the ventricle.

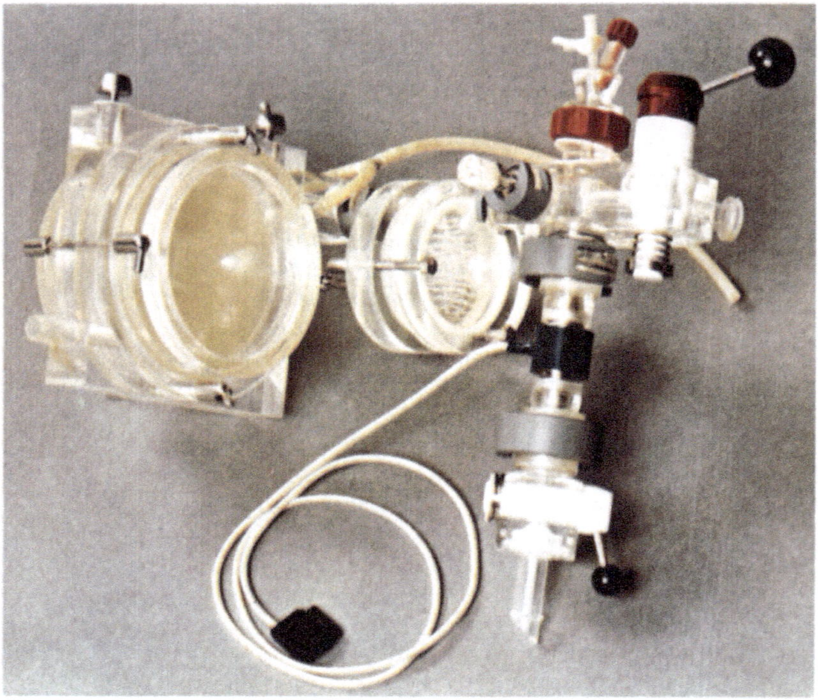

fig. 9

Proximal capillary resistor and compliance of a three part windkessel attached to the aortic cannula and central valve. The compliance consists of two air chambers separated from the blood by polyurethane membranes. Pressure inside the chambers is maintained at approximately arterial pressure level.

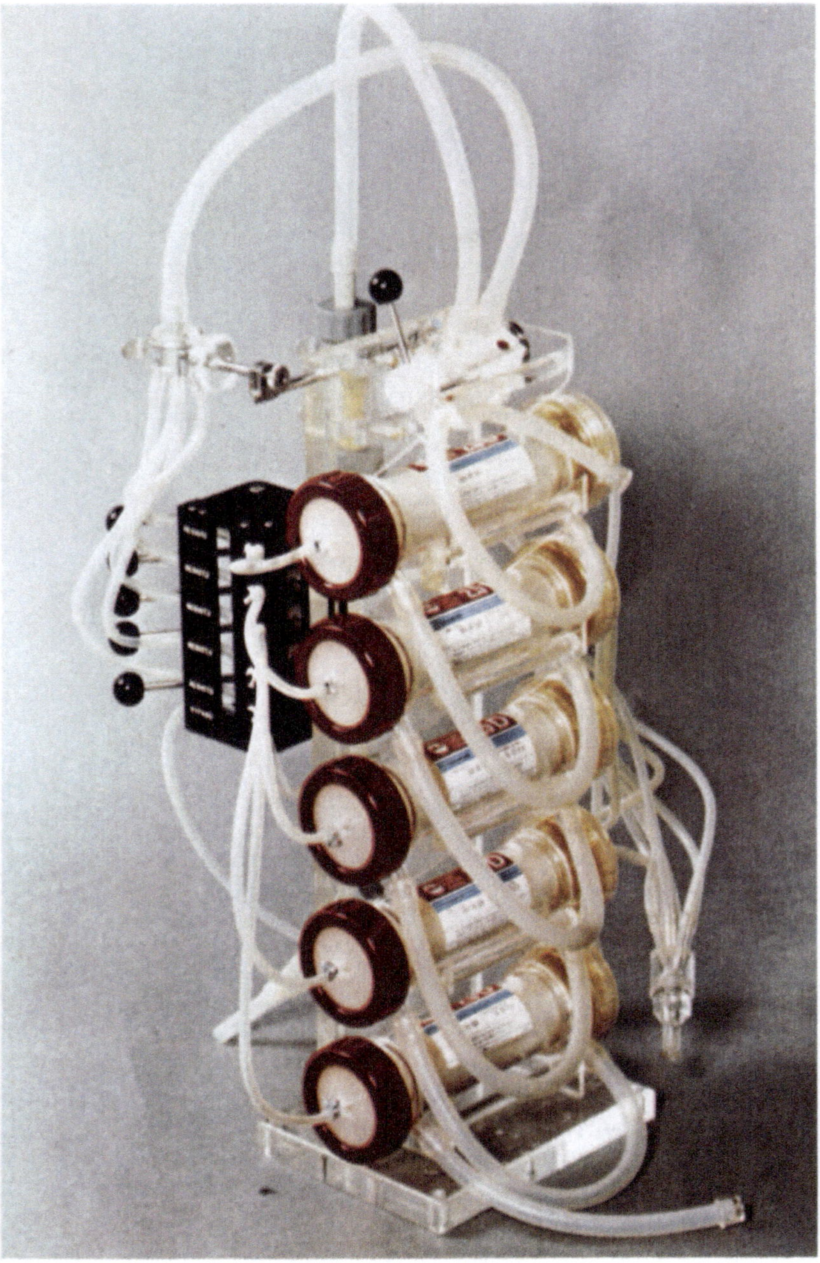

fig. 10

Distal resistor of the artificial haemodynamic impedance, made from five artificial kidneys (Cordis) in parallel. Switches serve to connect the kidneys either to the aorta or to a separate perfusion pump which maintains circulation when the kidneys are switched off. A two-way valve (on top) is used to bypass the system if required with a simple Starling resistor attached at the rear.

8 CORONARY FLOW AND OXYGEN CONSUMPTION

Using the right heart bypass technique, total coronary flow and oxygen saturation in the mixed coronary venous blood can be measured and oxygen consumption of the heart can be calculated. Results can be verified by measuring oxygen uptake from the respiratory gas mixture, using Starling's method[20]. In a healthy preparation at 38° C, coronary flow is about 70 ml/min/100 g heart tissue. When the left atrial pressure is set at +1 mmHg, and the mean aortic, pressure at 60 mmHg, venous saturation varies between 35 and 45% and oxygen consumption measures 8-10 ml/min/100 g. Coronary venous saturation and flow are a sensitive indicator of the condition of the coronary system and the myocardium. Mechanical damage to the heart inevitably causes an increase of venous saturation and flow, which increase is only partly reversible.

Left atrial pressure influences on oxygen consumption of the heart are far more pronounced than those of aortic pressure. A rise of left atrial pressure of only 4 mmHg in the proper pressure range will double oxygen uptake, while an increase of mean aortic pressure from 40 to 140 mmHg at constant left atrial pressure raises oxygen consumption only with about 20 per cent. The pronounced effect of end-diastolic dimensions on oxygen consumption undoubtedly results both from an increase in wall stress developed at the same systolic pressure and from changes in the mean value and in the distribution of initial fibre lengths in the myocardium. At a given initial fibre length the costs, in terms of oxygen consumption, of developing isometric tension followed by some degree of shortening are considered to be slightly less than the costs of pure, isometric tension development.

It will be difficult, however, to prove this in an intact heart preparation. Even when left atrial pressure is rigidly kept constant, the end-diastolic shape of the ventricle and even end-diastolic pressure varies with aortic pressure. The study of aortic pressure influences on oxygen demand therefore requires an elaborate technique for controlling left ventricular end-diastolic dimensions instead of simply left atrial mean pressure. Another problem is that the degree of shortening of ventricular fibers increases when aortic pressure is decreased in a non-linear fashion. Shortening of ventricular fibers is minimal but not completely absent when the aorta is cross-clamped, when aortic pressure is lowered a maximal degree of shortening is already reached at a pressure of about 60-70 mmHg, when the ejection fraction reaches its maximal value. The geometry of the ventricles thus prevents any further increase of fiber shortening when aortic pressure is reduced further. It would therefore be unlikely that oxygen consumption measured at constant end-diastolic dimensions decreases proportionally with aortic pressure over the entire pressure range. Anyhow, the influence of aortic pressure on oxygen demand in an heart-lung preparation and measured under fixed initial load conditions, is considerably smaller than in the intact organism where ventricular filling pressure is allowed to increase when arterial pressure rises.[18].

Heart rate is another factor known to influence oxygen uptake profoundly in the intact organism. In an isolated heart-lung preparation in which left aterial pressure is kept constant the effect of heart rate is far less pronounced. An increase in heart rate above its normal resting value in such a preparation is met by a reduction of stroke volume, cardiac output as a result is usually maintained at an approximately constant level. The reduction of stroke volume partly compensates for the increase in heart rate and oxygen consumption increases very little or not at all when heart rate is increased from 120 to 200 per minute. The effect of heart rate on oxygen consumption is however also influenced by aortic pressure. At high arterial pressures above 100 mmHg mean pressure oxygen uptake increases more steeply with heart rate. The effects on oxygen uptake of an increase in heart rate beyond 200 per minute are less predictable. Measurements are complicated in this range because end-diastolic dimensions may vary even when mean left atrial pressure is constant. The study of the effects of high heart rates therefore requires control of left ventricular dimensions instead of left atrial pressure.

Oxygen consumption studies on isolated hearts can only be interpreted in terms of pressure development and fibre shortening if the metabolic conditions of the preparation are well-known. A shift from aerobic glucose breakdown to metabolism of free fatty acids changes the efficiency of the preparation, which complicates the interpretation considerably. In the heart-lung preparation perfused with whole blood it usually takes about one hour before metabolism is based on glucose breakdown. Stored fat is probably not metabolized in an appreciable quantity after one hour of perfusion if glucose is provided in sufficient concentration. This may not be true when the fat content of the tissue is abnormally high, and also not when catecholamines are added to the circulating blood. Especially studies on catecholamine effects on oxygen demand requires additional information on glucose consumption derived from consecutive measurements of glucose concentration.

Coronary flow is up to a great extent determined by the oxygen demand of the myocardial tissue. The increase of oxygen uptake with left atrial pressure between −1 to +2 mmHg is reflected in an increase of coronary flow while venous oxygen saturation decreases slightly. The flow increase is medicated by the autoregulatory properties of the coronary vascular bed. The dynamic range of coronary autoregulation shifts to a higher level if oxygen demands are increased, thereby increasing flow at the same aortic pressure. Coronary flow is in addition influenced by both aortic and left atrial pressure directly. When aortic pressure rises coronary flow increases beyond the value needed to meet the increased oxygen demand. Venous saturation therefore increases when aortic pressure is raised. Surprisingly left atrial pressure exerts an opposite effect on coronary flow. This becomes evident above 3 mmHg when oxygen demand increases only little when left atrial pressure is further increased. In this pressure range coronary flow decreases, while oxygen consumption is maintained by decreasing oxygen saturation of the coronary venous blood. The aortic pressure effect is the result of an imperfect coronary autoregulation, which fails to maintain an exactly constant flow for the full aortic pressure range.
The mechanism of the left atrial pressure effect is not clear. It may be releated to an effect of diastolic wall tension on coronary flow.

REFERENCES

1 **Baan J., P.L.M. Kerkhof, R.A. Moene, J. Rohmer and M.A.M. Giesberts**
Controlled perfusion of the coronary arteries in the experimental study of ventricular dynamics.
Int. Conf. on Cardiovascular Dynamics, Abstract no. 6 (1976)
Exerpta Medica Amsterdam/Oxford

---

2 **Carmeliet E., R. Xhonneux, A. van Glabbeek and R. Reneman**
Electrophysiological effects of Droperidol in different cardiac tissues.
Naunijn-Schmiedeberg's Arch. Pharmacol.Vol 293: 57-66 (1976)

---

3 **Duvelleroy M.A., M. Duruble, J.L. Martin, B. Teisseire, J. Droulez and M. Cain**
Blood-perfused working isolated rat heart.
J. Appl. Physiol. Vol 41: 603-607 (1976)

---

4 **Eisels J.H., J.A. Reitan, M. Torten and C.H. Miller**
Myocardial sparing effect of Fentanyl during halothane anesthesia in dogs.
Br. J. Anesth. Vol 47: 937-940 (1975)

---

5 **Elzinga G.**
Cross talk between left and right heart.
Ph. D. Thesis, Free University Amsterdam (1972)

---

6 **Hintze T.H. and G. Kaley**
Prostaglandins and the control of blood-flow in the canine myocardium.
Circ. Res. Vol 40: 313-320 (1977)

---

7 **Kadowitz P.J. and A.L. Hyman**
Influence of a prostaglandin endoperoxide analogue on the canine pulmonary vascular bed.
Circ. Res. Vol 40: 282-287 (1977)

8 **Knowlton F.P. and E.H. Starling**
The influence of variations in temperature and blood-pressure on the performance of isolated mammalian heart.
J. Physiology Vol 44: 206-219 (1912)

---

9 **Langendorff O.**
Untersuchungen am überlebenden Säugetierherzen.
Arch. Gesamte Physiol. Vol 61: 291-332 (1895)

---

10 **Markwalder J. and E.H. Starling**
A note on some factors which determine the blood-flow through the coronary circulation.
J. Physiol. Vol 47: 275-285 (1913)

---

11 **Neely J.R., H. Liebermeister, E.J. Battersby and H.E. Morgan**
Effect of pressure development on oxygen consumption by isolated rat heart.
Am. J. Physiol. Vol 212: 804-812 (1967)

---

12 **Newell Martin H.**
Studies from the Biol. Lab. of the John Hopkins University II, pp. 119 (1881): A new method for studying the mammalian heart.

---

13 **Patschke D., J.W. Gethmann, W. Hess, J. Tarnow and H. Waibel**
Effect of high dosages of Fentanyl and piritramide upon haemodynamics, coronary blood flow and myocardial oxygen consumption.
Anesthesist Vol 25: 309-317 (1976)

---

14 **Patterson S.W. and E.H. Starling**
The carbohydrate metabolism of the isolated heart-lung preparation.
J. Physiology Vol 47: 137-148 (1913)

---

15 **Patterson S.W. and E.H. Starling**
On the mechanical factors which determine the output of the ventricles.
J. Physiology Vol 48: 357-379 (1914)

16 **Sarnoff S.J., E. Braunwald, G.H. Welch, R.B. Case, W.N. Stainsby and R. Macruz**
Hemodynamic determinants of oxygen consumption of the heart with special reference to the tension-time index.
Am. J. Physiol. Vol 192(I): 148-156 (1958)

---

17 **Simaan J. and G. Fawaz**
The mechanical efficiency of the Starling heart-lung preparation.
Pflügers Archiv Vol 302: 123-132 (1968)

---

18 **Sonnenblick E.H., J. Ross and E. Braunwald**
Oxygen consumption of the heart. Newer concepts of its multifactorial determination.
Am. J. Cardiology Vol 22: 328-336 (1968)

---

19 **Spach M.S. and R.C. Barr**
Ventricular intramural and epicardial potential distributions during ventricular activation and repolarization in the intact dog.
Circ. Res. Vol 37: 243-257 (1975)

---

20 **Starling E.H. and M.B. Visscher**
The regulation of the energy output of the heart.
J. Physiol. Vol 62: 243-261 (1926)

---

21 **Steiner C. and T.W. Kovalik**
A simple technique for production of chronic complete heart blocks in dogs.
J. Appl. Physiol. Vol 25: 631-632 (1968)

---

22 **Westerhof N., G. Elzinga and P. Sipkema**
An artificial arterial system for pumping hearts.
J. Appl. Physiol. Vol 31: 776-781 (1971)

Additional information of this book
*(The Isolated Heart-Lung Preparation;
978-90-247-2107-8_OSFO)* is provided;

EXTRA MATERIALS extras.springer.com

http://Extras.Springer.com

GPSR Compliance

The European Union's (EU) General Product Safety Regulation (GPSR) is a set of rules that requires consumer products to be safe and our obligations to ensure this.

If you have any concerns about our products, you can contact us on ProductSafety@springernature.com

In case Publisher is established outside the EU, the EU authorized representative is:

Springer Nature Customer Service Center GmbH
Europaplatz 3
69115 Heidelberg, Germany

Batch number: 10682325

Printed by Printforce, the Netherlands